# "My Dad's Lungs from Smoking"

## J. Michael Hall

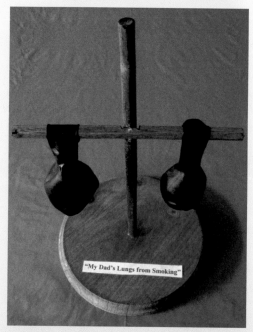

"My Dad's Lungs from Smoking"

### Ready to "Kick Your Smoking Habit"

### Ready for a "New Beginning"

### Start Fresh "One Simple Plan for One Tough Mission"

AuthorHouse™
1663 Liberty Drive
Bloomington, IN 47403
www.authorhouse.com
Phone: 833-262-8899

Because of the dynamic nature of the Internet, any web addresses or links contained in this book may have changed since publication and may no longer be valid. The views expressed in this work are solely those of the author and do not necessarily reflect the views of the publisher, and the publisher hereby disclaims any responsibility for them.

Any people depicted in stock imagery provided by Getty Images are models, and such images are being used for illustrative purposes only.
Certain stock imagery © Getty Images.

This book is printed on acid-free paper.

ISBN: 978-1-4567-6550-7 (sc)

Library of Congress Control Number: 2011906237

Print information available on the last page.

Published by AuthorHouse  02/27/2023

**author**HOUSE®

## My Dad's Lungs from Smoking
By J. Michael Hall

# *PREFACE*

As a former smoker, I am often asked to share my secret to finally "kicking the habit." Like many of you, I tried several different strategies that were supposed to help me stop smoking cigarettes and cigars, but all of my attempts were unsuccessful. It was only after all of the right ingredients were in place that I had the perfect recipe for quitting. Of course, since discovering a plan that actually worked, I have wanted to share it with the world!

Over the past 30 years since I quit smoking, I have become much more conscious and aware of others who smoke, especially young adults. On many occasions, it was all I could do not to take smokers by the shoulders and give them a good shake, trying to make them understand the consequences of what they are doing to their health, future, and, most importantly, loved ones. Afterwards, I would remind myself that these smokers were just like me. Like them, I started smoking because I thought it was "cool." I was convinced that I could quit any time I wanted and on my own terms. Sound familiar??

Recently, which seldom happens to me, I got a bad cold. I know this will sound gross, but while coughing up mucus, I noticed it was CLEAR. Wow! I then realized that when I smoked, the same mucus used to be BLACK! At that moment, all the frustration that had been building up inside me over the last 30 years finally surfaced, and I knew it was time to tell the world my story.

A couple of months ago, I became conscious of the number of emails I was getting on easy methods to stop smoking. Out of curiosity, I looked at some of the ads. Then after reading them, it hit me: they are costly and can have very dangerous side effects. My method is free with no side effects.

Smokers: what you're doing is terribly wrong! It is not "cool"! You cannot quit as easily as you think, and it's finally time for you to bite the bullet—like I did 30 years ago. Therefore, if you're ready, my three-step method will hopefully inspire you to a fresh start and a new beginning on life. Before long, you too will be able to say to your cigarettes and/or cigars...

**"I WIN...YOU LOSE."**

# THE BEGINNING, BEFORE THE "BEING COOL" MISTAKE

Before I share with you my simple plan to quit smoking, I thought I would give you a little background on myself. I think it's important because we all have similar characteristics. Like me, you were born into this world and the furthest thing from your mind was smoking that first cigarette.

While I go by Michael, my birth name is Jay Michael Hall. As the story goes, from my grandmother's diary, I was born on Tuesday, April 22, 1947 in Cleveland, Ohio. During the final stages of her pregnancy, my mother Dolores stayed in Cleveland with my father's mother. My father, Jay, continued to work in Youngstown, traveling back and forth until I was born.

My mother was taken to the hospital on April 22nd at 1:30 pm, and I was born later that day at 5:50 pm weighing in at 6 lbs and 14 oz. My father was able to make it to the hospital in time for my birth. However, due to complications with the delivery, my mother and I had to stay in the hospital until Wednesday, April 30th. On that day, we arrived at my grandmother's in an ambulance and she and my aunt Mary Jane put us to bed. My grandmother described the day we came home from the hospital: "They were both fine and we were all glad to have them home." In addition, as she wrote in her diary, "It rained all day until she and the baby were home and resting in bed, and then the sun came out."

I bet if you could go back to the time you were born, you would have a similar beginning. If we only knew what was in store down the road!

I was eventually followed by my three sisters, Rebecca, Kathleen, and Patricia, and my brother Gary. We were all brought up in Poland, Ohio, just outside of Youngstown. We were very fortunate to have a truly wonderful upbringing by our mom and dad. All through grade school, middle school, and high school, I participated in every activity I could, but I especially thrived in football and track. During those wonderful years, cigarettes were the furthest thing from my mind.

On June 9, 1965, I graduated from Poland Seminary High School. At that point, I was on top of the world and about to enter Youngstown State University. Things could not have been better until I went to our high school graduation party in Canfield, Ohio. Unbeknownst to me, my innocent world was about to fall apart.

## THE "BEING COOL" MISTAKE

As I mentioned, I attended my high school graduation party and had an unbelievably great time. That is, until I decided to "be cool" and smoke a cigarette. If only I had stopped after choking on that first puff, everything would have been fine. But no, I had to have a couple more, and because I continued to be on top of the world, I was well on my way to being sucked in and hooked on cigarettes.

During that summer, I left with my good friend on a three-month trip to New Jersey. By the end of the trip, I was smoking a pack a day. Even though my mother smoked and my father had quit years earlier, it was still very difficult to fess up and let them know I was now a smoker, too. I'll never forget the day I finally confessed about my new habit. "Don't worry, it's just a phase in my life and I can quit anytime I want."

Since they both smoked, there wasn't much for them to say, so they both just smiled and said almost together, "Right." I didn't realize at the time just how foolish I was to think I could quit on my terms. Twenty-nine years later I was still smoking cigarettes and cigars. Is this starting to sound familiar to you?

I smoked all the way through college and well into my 39 years of employment with Whirlpool Corporation, the greatest company in the world. I'll never forget one major event in my life that should have made me quit. Back in college, I had my first date with the girl who would eventually become my wife. When I picked up Henrietta (Henri for short) Caruso, I had a pack of Lucky Strikes in my pocket. I didn't think much about it until I had to use the restroom, which was in the basement where her father's business was located. Much to my surprise there were "no smoking" signs all over the place. I later asked her the purpose of the signs and she replied, "My parents are allergic to cigarette smoke."

I was trying very hard to make a good impression on the Caruso family, and since I was raised to be a good, polite, Catholic boy, I decided never to smoke around them. Before long, I was known as the boy who didn't smoke or drink. I finally had to set the record straight that I *did* drink, but I never had the heart to tell them that I smoked as well. I must have made a good impression after all. Just five years later, in 1971, Henri and I were married. However, I never smoked around her parents. Can you believe they both passed away without knowing my secret?! You would think that would've been reason enough to quit. Wrong!!

In 1975, Henri gave birth to our first child, Stephen. During the next eight years, we had two more sons, Jonathan and Patrick. I always loved telling people about "my three sons." As the years went by and they got older, smoking was still very prevalent in our society. Naturally, I wanted to warn them of the dangers of smoking, but it's difficult when you can't practice what you preach!

Around the mid to late '80s, we were receiving more information on the dangers of smoking and I knew it was time to quit. Besides my health and future, I wanted to quit for my family. I never smoked in the house or around my wife's family, but obviously that had no bearing on my attempts at quitting.  I soon began hearing on a continual basis from Henri and the boys "Dad, when are you going to stop smoking? When you're dead?!"

I remember one occasion when five of my coworkers and I decided we would quit together. We drove my new conversion van to a hypnotist more than three hours away, in Illinois. While I drove, the rest of the group smoked, played cards, and had a grand old time in the roomy van. We must have smoked 10 packs on the trip over to the hypnotist's office! I remember looking out the side mirror and watching the smoke literally pour out of the windows. After we were hypnotized, we drove back, stopped at a restaurant to eat, and had a beer together without smoking. However, within two to three weeks, we were all back on the cigarettes.

There finally came a time when those who smoked at Whirlpool could only smoke in designate areas. In our building, it was a small room in the basement. Today, as you might well know, this applies to almost all business establishments. Anyways, the smoke got so bad in the tiny room that we all chipped in and installed an exhaust fan. However, before we knew it, smoking was banned from all buildings, which meant we could only smoke in our cars. I felt like a sneak and started to drive around the block so no one would see me. Yes, just like I was sneaking with my wife's family. With all of this going on, the handwriting was on the wall, and I really knew it was time to quit.

For the next five years, I tried several different methods of quitting. Not only were they expensive, many of them also had serious side effects. What was I thinking? Do these sound familiar? Remember the experiences with Nicorette gum, the famous patch, cold turkey, electronic smokeless cigarettes, and various types of quit-smoking pills? Don't forget all the other aids that allowed you to continue smoking until the urge went away. Well, you guessed it, after all these attempts; I was still smoking cigarettes and cigars five years later. When I coughed, my mucus was **BLACK**, but still I didn't have the willpower to quit. While the doctors were suggesting that it was time, I didn't have a medical condition that made it a matter of life or death.  All I had was a bunch of self imposed excuses as to why I should not quit.

Like you, I found it extremely difficult—if not impossible—to stop smoking. I think the main reason I found quitting to be so troublesome was that I really, really enjoyed smoking, especially with that morning cup of coffee or a beer after a long day at work. However, I am now convinced I was lacking a **COMPELLING REASON** that hits you like a ton of bricks to quit.

I bet by now you have found some similarities between us and are thinking, "Even though I enjoy smoking, I really want to quit, too!"  Believe it or not, statistics indicate that nearly 70% of smokers want to quit.  It is not easy, and don't let anybody try to convince you otherwise. However, as you read on, I hope the knowledge of my success will **INSPIRE** you and give you the **WILL POWER** to finally kick your habit.

# STEP 1: A COMPELLING REASON TO QUIT

As I mentioned before, I really didn't have a compelling reason that made me want to quit. However, that all changed on March 3, 1994. As you go through life, there are certain events about which you remember specific details—including where you were when it happened and how you reacted. Events like the JFK, MLK, and RFK assassinations, the space shuttle Challenger accident, and 9/11, to name a few. Well, I have added March 3 and March 8, 1994 to my memory bank.

As I can remember, Thursday, March 3, 1994 was a somewhat rainy day with a temperature around 40 degrees. I got home from work a little early at around 5 pm and was talking with Henri while she was preparing dinner. Even though it was rainy and chilly, we were both feeling good about the week. The boys were expected home soon, so we could have dinner together as usual. Stephen was a senior at Lakeshore High School, Jonathan was in eighth grade at the middle school, and Patrick was in fifth grade at the elementary school.

All of a sudden, I heard the front door open and slam as Patrick arrived home. This was not the usual way he entered our home. It was as if he had something serious on his mind. I remember standing in the kitchen as he walked in holding something in his hand. He looked at me and then slammed the object on the kitchen table. I'll never forget what he said about his fifth-grade science project, as it was now sitting on the table. "Dad, this has been at the school for a week, and if this does not get you to stop smoking, nothing will."

He then left the room and went upstairs. While we never really talked about it again, I was naturally in shock. Henri and I were looking at his science project in complete awe. While looking at me and saying nothing, her eyes said it all: "Well, what are you going to do about it?"

Much to my surprise, Patrick's project below was very simple but really struck a nerve. He had taken a piece of wood in the shape of a circle with a small hole in the middle. There were two dowel rods in the shape of a cross. The bottom of the cross was placed in the hole in the circle. On each side of the cross hung two ugly, shriveled up black balloons. The caption across the piece of wood was "My Dad's Lungs from smoking." wow! how would you like to be presented with something like that from your child, family, or friend?

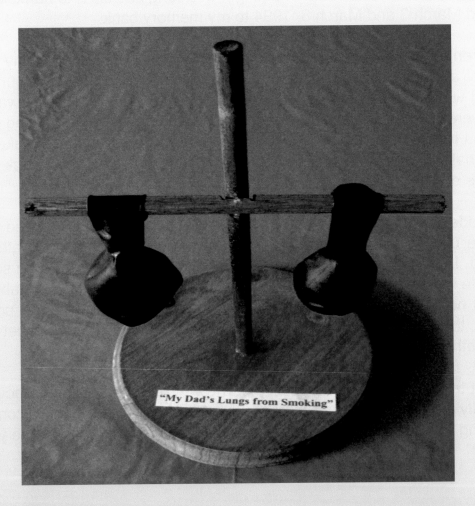

"My Dad's Lungs from Smoking"

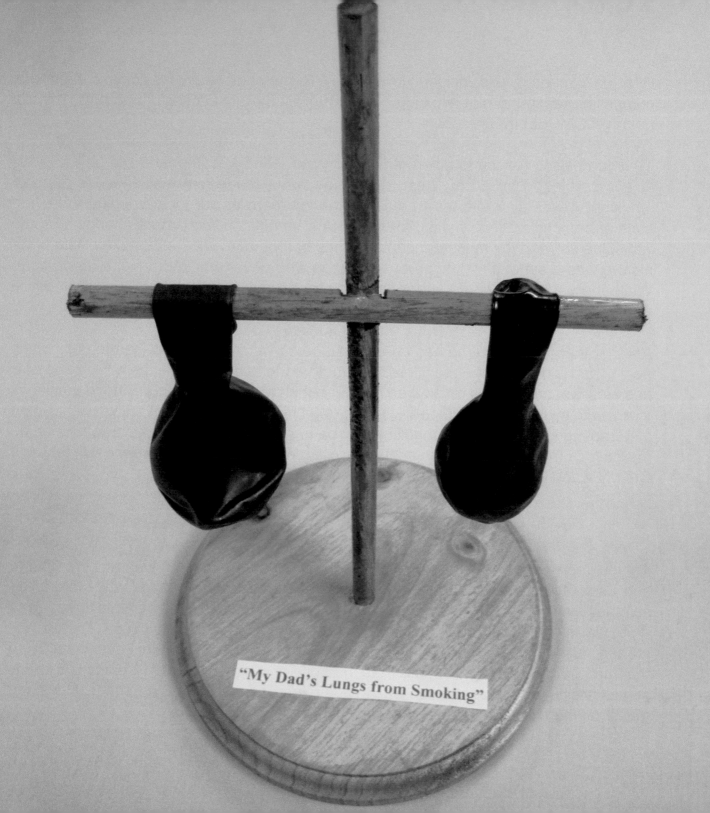

"My Dad's Lungs from Smoking"

Why do I mention this incident in my life? Remember when I said you needed a compelling reason to quit smoking? Well, after all the unsuccessful attempts, I finally got my COMPELLING reason.

That compelling reason is different for everyone. Mine just happened to be my son's science project. I asked my best friend, Joe, what made him quit after 20 years of smoking. It was a simple trip to the emergency room at our local hospital for a bad case of bronchitis. While waiting for the doctor, he noticed two pictures hanging on the wall. One showed the messed-up black lungs of a person who had smoked. The other picture was a set of pink lungs from a person who never smoked a cigarette or cigar. While there were no words under the pictures, he quit the next day. **Think about which lungs might be yours.**

Another friend found out he had an early-stage cancer and was advised to quit, which he did, and is now cancer free. However, another friend did not take the advice and now has emphysema. She is on oxygen for the rest of her life. The bottom line to quitting is that you really need that compelling reason that hits you like a ton of bricks, rather than just wanting to quit. If your compelling reason has not yet surfaced, feel free to imagine my science fair cross sitting in your living room. **Wow, think about that science fair project!!!** Cut out if you want!!!!

# STEP 2: SET THE DATE

As you know by now, I made several serious attempts to quit smoking and was never successful. I now had a compelling reason but needed to understand why I had failed so many times in the last five years of trying to quit. I knew that quitting "cold turkey" was a popular method, but I had tried it on several occasions with no success. Therefore, I started to ask myself "why?" Then I realized I had no criteria or goals associated with that method. Since I knew I had a reason to quit and did not want to be a failure to my son or family, my only alternative was to again try the "cold turkey" approach. However, this time, there had to be an objective, which is set forth below:

*"Successfully quit smoking cigarettes and cigars by selecting an easy to remember 'stop smoking' date by December 31, 1994."*

Well, it was early 1994. My son's project was still fresh, and with my goal in mind, I needed to quickly set a date. While all this was going through my mind, I knew the date had to be one that I could easily recall on a moment's notice. Thinking to myself, my brother's birthday was March 8, my son Steve was graduating from high school in 1994, and Jon's athletic jersey number was 23. *Therefore, on March 8, 1994, at Exit 23 on I-94, I threw out my last pack of cigarettes.*

You don't have to get that elaborate in selecting your date. *However, the key to success is to stop on a date that instinctively comes to your mind when you have that sudden urge to smoke.*

Many people told me if I quit I would gain weight. I don't know why, but I started sucking on Werther's Original hard candies every time I got the urge to smoke. That practice not only helped control my passion to smoke but got me through the whole ordeal without over-eating. After 30 years, I have gained only 10 lbs. Just a little tip I thought I would pass along…

I found setting the date to be extremely profound since this is not an easy thing you will be attempting to conquer. For a while, the urge will be constantly on your mind, especially during the first 72 hours. The six-month milestone is the most critical, as that is when the majority of people fail. Unfortunately, this is something you just have to overcome. You must keep telling yourself, "I made it another day." Before you know it, you will be one day, one week, one month, six months, one year, five years, 10 years, etc, into your objective. As time marches on, the urges become fewer and fewer. You just have to remember that one puff means you have to start all over from day one.

Imagine, you have quit for six months and something happens and you get the urge to just puff or smoke one cigarette. Guess what? If you did not think about your date and had that smoke, you must now start over with a new date. You will then ask yourself, "Was that smoke worth undoing all your efforts over the last six months?" In other words, when you get that urge to smoke, simply think of your date and instantly remember your accomplishments. Hopefully, that will deter you from lighting up.

Since I quit smoking on my brother's birthday, I continue to send him a card every year wishing him a happy birthday—with one extra line. This year it read, "Gary, it has been 30 years." With that in mind, I truly do not want to start over. Sadly, I continually hear people say they have quit and then that one event occurs and they start back again. That is when you need that compelling reason and date to just say **NO!!!**

After all these years, I still get the feeling that it would be great to have a cigarette, especially as I'm writing this book. I don't think the desire ever goes away. However, when those urges occur, March 8, 1994 pops in my mind, reminding me of how long it has been and that starting over is not an option.

Good luck setting your date.

## STEP 3: THE 12-MONTH FOLLOW-UP RULE

As we have previously discussed, my method may be simple, but the task at hand is not. Quite by accident, I stumbled on to the importance of the 12-month follow-up, which is the final step to help ensure your success.

On April 8, 1994, I had quit smoking for 30 days and was feeling pretty darn proud of my accomplishment. There were some times when I wanted a smoke, but I continued to remember my date and suck on my Werther's Original hard candies.

After a month, I decided to finally go to a smoking establishment, as I could not avoid them for the rest of my life. I wanted to test my **"Compelling Reason and Set the Date"** steps by having a beer with all that smoke and excitement around me. Much to my surprise, I had a great time and did not smoke one cigarette. My objective was coming closer and closer to becoming a reality and I felt great.

When I arrived home that night, I was in total shock! For the first time in 29 years, I wreaked of smoke. I never realized what I smelled like and finally understood why everyone wanted me to quit. I don't know if I was just embarrassed or disgusted with myself for what I had been doing to not only my health but, to anyone that came around me. I remember this as though it was yesterday. My clothes smelled so bad that I hung them in the garage for the night rather than bringing them inside the house. Think about it. Has anyone ever told you how bad you smell? Whether you want to believe me or not, they are right!!! You just have to experience it to know what they're talking about. Even today, I can tell when I am around a smoker.

The next day, I went back and revised my objective, set forth below, and step three was born:

*"Successfully quit smoking cigarettes and cigars by selecting an easy to remember 'stop smoking' date, to include 12 monthly visits to a smoking establishment, by December 31, 1994."*

Therefore, 30 days after your last cigarette and/or cigar, visit a smoking establishment. Continue your visits once a month for the next 12 months. This will reassure you that you made the right choice. I only wish I could be there to hear your thoughts when you smell your clothes after that first visit!

In my case, it only took about three visits—even though I continued for the full 12 months—to realize it is really not cool to smoke. I knew I had made the right decision to quit.

Good luck with your monthly follow-up visits to your local smoking establishment.

# THE "STATISTICS" THAT SHOULD GET YOUR ATTENTION

Now that we have covered the three steps, I would like you to review some startling statistics. These should prove helpful and offer some additional incentives as to why you need to set a date, once you realize you do have a compelling reason to quit.

As you no doubt already know, the link between cigarette smoking and cancer, heart disease, and various breathing problems has been well established for many years. More importantly, quitting reduces these risks almost as soon as you stop smoking. I know you have seen some of the figures before, but I want you to take a serious look and not simple shrug them off. Since I have been in your shoes, I know you do not think they apply to you. However, now that I have quit, I understand that they indeed applied to me and to you as well.

My intent is not to flood you with a bunch of statistics, but there are some that you really need to think about. Take your time and study some eyebrow-raising statistics, set forth below, from Healthy Living, American Nonsmokers' Rights Foundation, MSN Money, and Healthline.

**Effects of smoking**: (Healthy Living)

- Worldwide-tobacco use is responsible for more than 5 million deaths. Annual and current trends indicate deaths will start to exceed 8 million each year.
- In the United State alone, it is estimated that more than 43 million adults are smokers. That is nearly 20% of the population that is over the age of 18.
- 22.3% are male smokers.
- 17.4% are female smokers
- For every person who dies from a smoking related disease, 20 more suffer from at least one serious illness related to smoking.
- Nearly 50,000 nonsmokers die annually from secondhand smoke exposure.

- Even with all the knowledge of the health hazards of smoking, each day, nearly 1,000 kids (peer pressure and the "being cool" effect) under the age of 18 and 1,800 adults (peer pressure, the "being cool" effect, and stress) 18 and over will start smoking on a daily basis.

Growing number of States banning smoking in general public places, as of 1/2/11: (American Nonsmokers' Rights Foundation)

- 79.4% of the US population lives under smoking bans in workplaces and/or restaurants and/or bars.
- A total of 23 states have a law in effect that requires workplaces, restaurants, and bars to be 100% smoke free. These laws, along with local laws in other states, protect 47.8% of the US population.
- A total of 29 states have a law in effect that requires restaurants and bars to be 100% smoke free. These laws, along with local laws in other states, protect 63.7% of the US population.
- A total of 16 states have enacted 100% smoke free laws for all state-regulated gaming.
- Bottom line, whether you like it or not, it is becoming harder and harder to smoke in public places. The driving force is the fact that 50,000 people die each year from secondhand smoke.

**Estimated annual cost to smoke cigarettes:** (MSN Money)

- The latest information indicates that the average cost for a pack of cigarettes is around $4.50 to $5, including taxes, depending on where you live.
- Using the lower number, a pack-a-day smoker burns through about $31.50 per week, or $1,638 per year.
- To estimate your cost, simply plug in what you pay per pack and the number of packs per day you smoke. You may be astounded at your yearly cost.

**What happens when you quit smoking?** You will be amazed, as I was, to see how your body responds, beginning just 20 minutes after you quit. (Healthline)

While I experienced these same effects on my body, I have added some of my own experiences that helped me to get through the ordeal.

- **20 minutes**: You will begin to feel good about your health and glad the date is finally set, as your heart rate will begin to drop back to normal.

- **2 hours**: Your heart rate and blood levels will have decreased to near healthy levels. However, the nicotine withdrawal symptoms will usually start. Don't trick yourself into smoking again just because you're feeling irritated. Now is the time to remember your date and why you quit. Start sucking on those Werther's Original hard candies. **You will make it!!!**

- **12 hours**: The carbon monoxide in your body decreases to normal levels and your blood-oxygen levels increase to normal.

- **24 hours**: While you're not out of the woods, your risk for a heart attack will have already begun to drop.

- **48 hours**: Your ability to smell and taste is enhanced. This illustrates why monthly visits to smoking establishments are so important! Previously, you had become immune to the odor of cigarette smoke.

- **72 hours**: The nicotine will be completely out of your body. The withdrawal will increase at this time. Again, don't trick yourself into smoking again just because you're feeling irritated. Remember why you quit, your date, and suck on those Werther's Original hard candies. **You will make it!!!**

- **2 to 3 weeks**: Your lungs will start to feel clear, and you'll start to breath easier.

- **1 to 9 months**: Your lungs will begin to regenerate and coughing and shortness of breath will decrease dramatically. Withdrawal symptoms will go away.

- **6 months:** **This is the most critical month**. Brain research shows that nicotine is powerfully addictive. Three out of four smokers who try to kick the habit relapse with-in six months. You have made it this far, so remember the reason you quit, your date, and make that six-month follow-up visit.

- **1 year:** **YAY!!!** Your risk of heart disease is lowered 50% compared to when you were smoking. Do not forget to follow up by going to a smoking establishment **See if you notice the smell of your clothes.**

- **5 years:** Your risk of a stroke is now the same as someone who never smoked **Congratulations!!!**

- **10 years**: Your risk of dying from lung cancer will drop to half of a smoker's.

- **15 years**: Your risk of heart disease will be back to the same level of someone who does not smoke.

- **30 years:** **This is where I am, and I feel GREAT!!!!**

The most important statistic that I want you to remember comes again from Healthy Living. As you formulate your thoughts to quit smoking or not, they report:

- Nearly 70% of smokers want to quit smoking altogether.
- Approximately 40% of smokers will try to quit.
- About 7% will succeed at quitting their first try. That may sound like a small number, but it is more than 3 million people.
- 3 to 4% of people who quit smoking will do it "cold turkey."

# SUMMARY

I hope you have enjoyed our conversation and have obtained some insights on what it takes to kick your habit.

Once again, the three steps that I used to quit "cold turkey" are set forth below:

## *STEP 1*

Remember, everyone has a reason to start smoking in the first place but you must have a **compelling reason** to quit. You'll have a better chance of success if that reason is constantly on your mind. In my case, I can remember Patrick slamming that science fair project on the kitchen table as though it were yesterday. The title, **"My Dad's Lungs from Smoking,"** was one powerful statement.

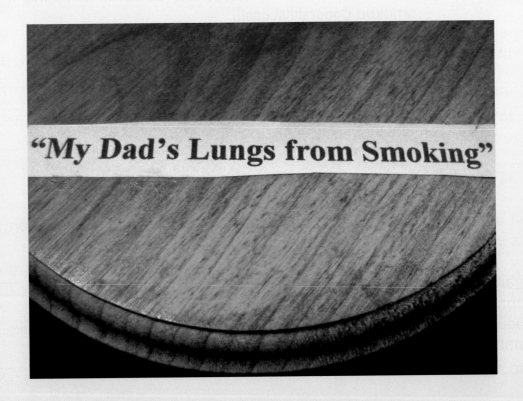

## STEP 2

**Set your date** and constantly keep it in the back of your mind. You need to instantly know how long you have been successful and that starting over is not an option. After 17 years, my date remains **March 8, 1994.**

## STEP 3

Perform those all-important **follow-up visits for 12 months**. While it is becoming more difficult to find smoking establishments, the casinos are normally a smoking environment. If for nothing more, the objective is to smell your clothes when you come home. Even after 30 years, I still follow up at smoking establishments and put my clothes in the garage for the night as I say **"Thank God I quit!"** when I walk back into the house.

After sharing my **One Simple Plan for One Tough Mission,** I feel a personal interest in your success, so please give it that good old-fashioned attempt to conquer your smoking addiction. Ask any smoker, including me; it is easy to start but hard to quit. In addition, remember to be aware of the statistics we reviewed, especially potential **DEATH** and, of course, the money you will save over the course of your non-smoking years. Those statistics played a major factor in giving me the added willpower to stick to my conviction when quitting "cold turkey."

Before you know it, you will have stopped on your own rather than through those ill-advised aids, such as gum or pills with potentially dangerous side effects. You will have done it for **FREE**. Just like me, you, too, will be able to say to your cigarettes and/or cigars, as I did 17 years ago:

**"I WIN...YOU LOSE."**

# Internet Sources

Smith, Hilary. "The high cost of smoking." <u>MSN.com.</u> September 3, 2008. January 20, 2011< <u>http://articles.moneycentral.msn.com/Insurance/InsureYourHealth/</u> <u>HighCostOfSmoking.aspx</u>

Wolfson, Elijah. "What Happens When You Quit Smoking?" <u>Healthline.com.</u> January 20, 2011< <u>http://www.healthline.com/health-slideshow/quit-smoking-timeline</u>

"Overview List: How many Smoke-free Laws?" <u>No Smoke.org.</u> January 2, 2011. February 10, 2011< <u>http://www.no-smoke.org/pdf/mediaordlist.pdf</u>

"Smoking Statistics/Quitting Smoking" <u>Quit Smoking. Pharmacy Discount rx.com.</u> February 10, 2011< <u>http://quitsmoking.pharmacydiscountrx.com/stats.html</u>

## Internet Sources

Ekhart, Hillary. "The high cost of smoking." USA.com. September 6, 2008. January 20, 2011 <http://usa.com/...>

Wilson, Elliot. "What Happens When You Quit Smoking?" Healthline.com. January 10, 2008 <http://www.healthline.com/health/...>

"However, Is It True, Maybe Smoke Are Free?" UK-Smoke.org. February 2, 2011 <http://www.uk-smoke.org/...>

"Immediate Statistics: Quitting Smoking." PharmacyDiscount.com. February 10, 2011 <http://www.pharmacydiscount.com/...>

Printed in the United States
by Baker & Taylor Publisher Services